YOUR KNOWLEDGE HAS VALUE

- We will publish your bachelor's and
  master's thesis, essays and papers

- Your own eBook and book -
  sold worldwide in all relevant shops

- Earn money with each sale

Upload your text at www.GRIN.com
and publish for free

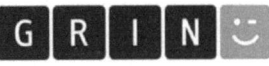

Bibliographic information published by the German National Library:

The German National Library lists this publication in the National Bibliography; detailed bibliographic data are available on the Internet at http://dnb.dnb.de .

This book is copyright material and must not be copied, reproduced, transferred, distributed, leased, licensed or publicly performed or used in any way except as specifically permitted in writing by the publishers, as allowed under the terms and conditions under which it was purchased or as strictly permitted by applicable copyright law. Any unauthorized distribution or use of this text may be a direct infringement of the author s and publisher s rights and those responsible may be liable in law accordingly.

Imprint:

Copyright © 2016 GRIN Verlag, Open Publishing GmbH
Print and binding: Books on Demand GmbH, Norderstedt Germany
ISBN: 9783668478725

This book at GRIN:

http://www.grin.com/en/e-book/370179/contraceptive-use-and-associated-factors-among-female-students-in-wolaita

Wesen Altaye

Contraceptive Use and Associated Factors among Female Students in Wolaita Sodo ATVET College, Southern Ethiopia

GRIN Publishing

GRIN - Your knowledge has value

Since its foundation in 1998, GRIN has specialized in publishing academic texts by students, college teachers and other academics as e-book and printed book. The website www.grin.com is an ideal platform for presenting term papers, final papers, scientific essays, dissertations and specialist books.

Visit us on the internet:

http://www.grin.com/

http://www.facebook.com/grincom

http://www.twitter.com/grin_com

Wolaita Soddo ATVET College

Contraceptive Use and Associated Factors among Female Students in Wolaita Sodo
ATVET College, Southern Ethiopia

By
Wesen Altaye Aydiko

A research submitted to Wolaita Soddo ATVET Colloge
Advisor:-Research team of the colloge

November, 2016
Wolaita Sodo, Ethiopia

Abstract

Background: Contraceptive use by sexually active female students in a College setting is both practical and intelligent. Reliable, consistent, and therapeutically correct contraceptive use prevents unintended pregnancies and assures a greater likelihood of uninterrupted or impeded higher education for the young woman.

Objectives: The objective of this study was to assess contraceptive use and identify the factors associated with contraceptive use.

Methods: An institutional based cross-sectional survey was conducted among 1067 female college students of Wolaita Soddo ATVET from October 21, 2016 to November 9, 2016. Multistage sampling technique with Probabilities proportional to size was used. After data collection, each questionnaire was checked for completeness and consistency. Data was analyzed by manually then different frequency tables, graphs and descriptive summaries were used to describe the study variables and 95% Confidence Intervals to adjust for possible confounding variables.

Results: Of the total respondents, 598(96.5 %) of them replied that they have heard about contraceptives. Among those who have ever heard of contraceptives, 221 (35.6 %) mentioned condom only, 155 (25.6 %) mentioned pills only and 149(24.0%) Norplant and 44(7.11%). This study has shown that 450 72(%) of the female college students use contraceptive.

Conclusion: ATVET collage clinic also has high contribution on contraceptive utilization by providing access to contraceptive with multiple chooses. The collage also creating Reproductive Health Clubs in the college and enhance the awareness on contraceptive

Acknowledgement

First and foremost, I would like to thank the research team of the college for their invaluable comments and suggestions throughout the proposal work.

My special thanks and sincere appreciation also go to Wolaita Soddo ATVET College administration and health center staff as well as supervisors and study participants for contribution to the success of the data collection.

Acronyms and Abbreviation

ATVET:	Agricultural Technical, vocational and Educational Training
EC:	Emergency contraception
ECPs:	Emergency contraceptive pills
ECs:	Emergency contraceptives
EDHS:	Ethiopian Demographic Health Survey
ESOG:	Ethiopian Society of Obstetrics and Gynecologists
FGAE:	Family Guidance Association of Ethiopia
FP:	Family Planning
GBV:	Gender based violence
IUCD;	Intra Uterine Contraceptive Device
MMR:	Maternal Mortality Rate
MOH;	Ministry of health
NRM:	natural resource management
RH:	Reproductive health
SDC:	Skill development center
SD;	Standard Deviation
WHO:	World Health Organization

Contents

List of table

List of figure

1. Introduction

In every setting, sexual activity appears to begin during adolescence among a substantial proportion of youth. Much of this activity is risky; the practice of contraception and condom use is often erratic and unwanted pregnancy and unsafe abortions are observed in many settings. Sexual relations are not always consensual: force and coercion are far from unknown. While young people tend to be generally well informed, they have only patchy in-depth knowledge of issues related to sexuality. Moreover, expressed norms often conflict with behavior. Moreover, there are wide gender-based differences in sexual conduct, and in the ability to negotiate sexual activity and contraceptive use. Contraceptive experience of abortion-seekers suggests that practice tends to be irregular, or incorrect, and the method of choice is largely traditional (1).

Adolescent pregnancy is common place in many countries. About 16 million adolescent girls aged 15-19 give birth each year, roughly 11% of all births worldwide. Almost 95% of these births occur in developing countries. Half of all adolescent births occur in just seven countries: Bangladesh, Brazil, the Democratic Republic of Congo, Ethiopia, Nigeria, India and the United States (2).

Young people disproportionately resort to unsafe abortion due to limited availability and high cost of quality medical abortion procedures and because they have more unwanted pregnancies than older women (3). Overall risk of death from unsafe abortion is by far the highest in Africa, where the case fatality rate reaches 7 deaths per 1000 unsafe abortions (4). Pregnancies occurring among unmarried women are often unintended.

Unintended pregnancies result from contraceptive non-use, misuse, and method failure. Adolescent women are more likely not to use and to misuse contraceptive than older women (5).

In Ethiopia where approximately 33% of the population falls between the ages of 10-24, a significant proportion of the youth practice unsafe sex and sex at early age (6, 7).

The Ethiopian Ministry of Health has developed of the national adolescent and youth reproductive health (AYRH) strategy, to alleviate the RH problem youth including the contraceptive needs (8). Furthermore, it has developed standards on youth friendly reproductive health services that entailed nine standards on how the service should be provided in different settings.

However, higher learning institutions, where only young people are residing, student clinics are not being utilized for contraceptive services. In spite of this, most of the existing services are non-youth friendly, undertaken in small scale and not well organized to meet the contraceptive service needs of this section of the population (9). Having this in mind this study tried to assess the prevalence of contraceptive use and identify the associated factors among female students in Wolaita Sodo ATVET College.

1.2 Statement of the Problem

Unplanned pregnancies among young women are a worldwide problem with social and economic repercussions for the unprepared young individual (10). A critical challenge in the global effort to reduce maternal mortality is the persistence of unsafe abortion as a result of unwanted pregnancy, which accounts for 13% of Pregnancy related deaths worldwide (11).

In many low income countries, the lack of knowledge about and access to Contraceptive Use may result in women resorting to unsafe abortions, which contribute significantly to maternal morbidity and mortality (12). Each year, about 210 million women around the world become pregnant. Among them, about 75 million pregnancies (36%) are unplanned and/or unwanted. And globally, more than 20 million women experience ill health as a result of pregnancy each year (13, 14). It is estimated that between 8 and 30 million pregnancies each year result from contraceptive failure either due to inconsistent or incorrect use of contraceptive methods or failure of the method itself (15). Research studies conducted in the USA have reported that higher rates of unintended pregnancy occur among college-age women, with 60% of pregnancies among 20-24 years old being unintended. The percentage of unintended pregnancy is even higher among 18-19-year-old females (79%) (16). Unintended pregnancy poses a major challenge to the reproductive health of young adults especially in developing counties. High rates of unintended pregnancy are associated with higher incidences of abortion, & specifically unsafe abortions, which further place women at risk of death and disability.

Each year, an estimated 19 million unsafe abortion occurs in the developing world, and around 70,000 women die from abortion –related causes where abortion is often legally restricted and maternal care services are lacking. In addition to those who die from unsafe abortions, tens of thousands suffer from chronic and sometimes irreversible health consequences, including infertility (11, 17).

Unsafe abortion is often the only option available to women who wish to terminate a Pregnancy in countries where abortion is illegal /legally restricted, or where significant access barriers exist including lack of access, Knowledge or awareness and use of contraception. By

5

expanding number of family planning's and increasing awareness's especially towards contraception options available to women is a critical part of increasing contraceptive coverage, decreasing unintended pregnancies and reducing maternal morbidity and mortality around the globe (18). Lack of use or access to contraceptives is a major cause of unwanted Pregnancy. More than half of all women in the developing world are at risk because they are using a traditional method with high failure rates; or they are using a reversible method that requires regulars supply; or they are using no method at all. Since no contraceptive work perfectly every time even wide spread modern contraceptive use will not completely eliminate the need for recourse to abortion (19).

Unsafe abortion as a result of unplanned/unwanted pregnancy is one of the leading causes of maternal mortality and morbidity in Ethiopia. Ethiopia has a high incidence of unwanted pregnancies and unsafe/septic abortions, particularly among adolescents. Several studies in the country have revealed that women who tend to undergo induced abortion are below the age of 30 years and are literate; many of whom being above the secondary educational level. Reasons for such huge numbers of unintended pregnancies in Ethiopia include a low rate of contraceptive use, method failure, and high unmet need for contraceptives (20).

In Ethiopia according to the survey conducted in 2000 by ESOG in nine administrative regions, 25.6 percent of 1075 abortion cases were induced abortions. Among them, 58 percent of the cases were in the age range 20-29 years. Of those pregnancies ended in abortion 60 percent were unplanned 50 percent were unwanted (21). Adolescent women face a high risk of unintended pregnancies and unsafe abortion, with devastating consequences for their lives and health (22).

According to the EDHS 2005, Ethiopia has one of the highest maternal mortality ratios in the world, estimated at 673 deaths per 100,000 live births. And in Ethiopia about 25,000 women die every year due to pregnancy and child birth complications, and several studies indicate that unsafe abortion may account for up to 25-35% of the maternal deaths in Ethiopia. Unplanned pregnancies are the result of various factors, including a lack of knowledge about menstruation and pregnancy, a lack of access to and knowledge about how to use contraceptives, difficulties in using contraceptives because of partner's or family objections; contraceptive failure and sexual assault (23).

Wider use of contraception could prevent a substantial proportion of the millions of unplanned pregnancies that occur every year. Safe and effective hormonal preparations are available that can prevent a pregnancy by inhibiting ovulation, altering the ability of sperm to fertilize an ovum or inhibiting implantation in the womb (24, 25). Hence, this study will try to explore Contraceptive Use and Associated Factors among Female Students in Wolaita Sodo ATVET College, Southern Ethiopia.

1.3. Significance of the Study

This study is needed because contraceptives play a vital role in preventing unwanted pregnancies, induced abortions. It also helps for those female college students to have knowledge about contraceptives from being interrupted their education as a result of unwanted pregnancy. Research on Contraceptive Use and Associated Factors among college students may help to inform policy makers and education planners in Ethiopia. Unfortunately, no tangible research has been conducted in this area among the college students in the town. This study is assumed to provide baseline data for policy makers and education planners in developing appropriate evidence-based strategies and curricula in college to prevent unintended pregnancy and will have a great role for nursing and midwifery in consolidating, scaling up and keep up of the achievement in the health sectors of Ethiopia.

2. Literature Review

Fertility is high in Ethiopia. Women have an average of 5.4 children during their lifetimes and these larger families' burden parents or caregivers in providing all that is needed for their proper care. Using contraceptives is an important step towards limiting family size. (26)

Contraceptive use in Ethiopia is not without socio-demographic predictors and cultural complexities. A variety of factors are associated with contraceptive use in the country. Major factors include marital status, educational level of wife, occupational status, family monthly income, and number of pregnancies, number of live births, number of living children, spousal educational level, and spousal occupational status. (27)

Unprotected intercourse can occur when there is coerced/ unplanned sex & when barrier methods break or dislodged or when other contraceptives are improperly used. Contraceptive Use prevents pregnancies. (28). The potential of Contraceptive Use and EC to prevent unwanted pregnancies and its utilization in developed counties has been well documented, However in vast majority of developing counties including Ethiopia the potential clients' service providers and the services status is not well documented. Regarding the knowledge that help the women to decide whether to use or not about Contraceptive Use there is a wide gap between developed & Non- developed nations even between nations of different area. Different studies showed non developed nation have very low awareness whereas developed have higher awareness. Among six different studies in Ethiopia from 24-85.5% had heard about Contraceptive Use and Emergency contraceptive, from the six knowledge assessment studies, four studies had less than 50% awareness and only two studies in Bahirdar and Jimma University had 83.5%and 53% awareness respectively. Other studies from other countries had relatively had more awareness. For instances, studies in san Francisco 89%, Katmandu - Nepal 68 %.(29)

A study done on Knowledge and practice of contraception among female undergraduates in the University of Lagos, Nigeria, revealed that 67.8% of the respondents reported knowing about emergency contraception. More than half (56.1%) were sexually active and of this group, 96.8% had ever practiced contraception with only 33.9% having ever practiced emergency contraception. However, only 37.8% and 36.3% of respondents who had reported knowing about contraception knew the correct time frame for effective use, and correctly identified contraceptives respectively. Among those who were aware of, and had used emergency contraception, 34.1% obtained their information from health care providers, while the larger majority obtained from friends. Knowledge and practice of emergency contraception was directly related to age, level of study, medical education, marital status, sexual activity, previous history of use of contraceptives and previous history of induced abortion. (30).Other similar Studies conducted on knowledge, attitude and practice towards Contraception and Fertility awareness among University Students in Kampala, Uganda, Makerere University showed that the mean age of the participants was 21 years. Less than half (45.1%) had ever heard about emergency contraceptive pills (ECPs).The most common sources of information about EC were friends (34%), media (24.8%) and schools (19.4%). The ever pregnancy rate was 3.4 percent and 42 percent were in a steady relationship of three or more months. The contraceptive ever-use rate was 14.5 percent. Among the users, the most common methods were condoms (48.9%) and withdrawal (23.4%).Other research conducted among Jimma university community high school students showed that, 64% of respondents heard about contraceptive where as studies among client seeking abortion at clinic had low awareness about Emergency contraception, which is only 13.5-14% of all the respondents heard about it (31). Reduction in unplanned pregnancies leads to lower abortion rates. It has been estimated that 43% of decline in abortions that took place between 1994 & 2000 in the United States was due to the increased availability of Contraception. (32)

Studies conducted in Addis Ababa University and Unity University College showed that 43.5% of the students said that they have heard about contraceptives. When asked about specific types of emergency contraceptives, among those who have ever heard of emergency contraceptives, 82.8% mentioned pills and 34.1% mentioned intrauterine contraceptive devices (IUCDs). About 53% of the students had positive attitude towards emergency contraceptives and only 4.9% respondents reported that they had used emergency contraceptive methods previously (33).

Similar other research conducted at Gondar University students indicated that 24.0 % thought that there are methods that can be used to prevent pregnancy when a woman had unprotected sex. Overall, 18.8% knew the correct methods of emergency contraception (pill or IUCD). Of those who mentioned pill as the only method of emergency contraception, 73.3% said the pill should be used within 72 hours after unprotected sex. Only one student used pill as emergency contraceptive. Students in the health field have 6.8 times higher knowledge on emergency contraception compared to students of FBE. Generally, there was an increasing trend in the knowledge of students when their age and year of study increases. Married or divorced students had 3.36 times higher knowledge when compared with never married students. (34)

2.2 Gender Based Violence in College Students

GBV is physical, mental or social abuse (including sexual violence) and act, attempted or threatened, done with some type of force, manipulation, or coercion & without the informed consent of the affected person/ survivor. Forms of gender based violence (GBV) include sexual violence, sexual abuse, sexual harassment, sexual exploitation, early or forced marriage, discrimination and female genital cutting. In a qualitative study by consortium of RH association (CORHA) in four universities in Ethiopia, female university students had reported they were harassed & raped both in and outside the university compasses.

In a school based survey among high school students in Addis Ababa & west Shewa prevalence of completed & attempted rape was 5% and 10% respectively. In similar study among high school students in Debark, North- west Ethiopia, sexual violence was reported by 65.3% of respondents. (35)

2.3 Importance of Contraception for Youth

Contraception involves methods of contraception used for preventing a pregnancy after unplanned or unprotected sexual intercourse. The concept appears appropriate for adolescents and students in higher institutions or those in vocational training who are engaged in sporadic and occasional sexual intercourse's. The need for emergency contraception is clearly demonstrated by the occurrence of unwanted or induced pregnancies. In populations where most women of reproductive age don't have access to contraception, unwanted / mistimed pregnancies occur frequently. Most victims of unwanted pregnancy are adolescents, who are expelled from school, often ending their formal education & the potential for future employment. For fear of being expelled from school, many adolescent girls resort to clandestine abortion, which often results in series complications or death.

Many adolescents are subjected to have sex sporadically, which makes contraceptive planning difficult. Other experience contraceptive failure & their failure rates may be higher than adults due to their in experience. No method of contraception is 100% effective. Furthermore, few peoples use their method perfectly every time they have intercourse thus demonstrating the need for an emergency backup method. Also many young women experience coerced sex, including rape. (31)

2.4 Conceptual Frame Work

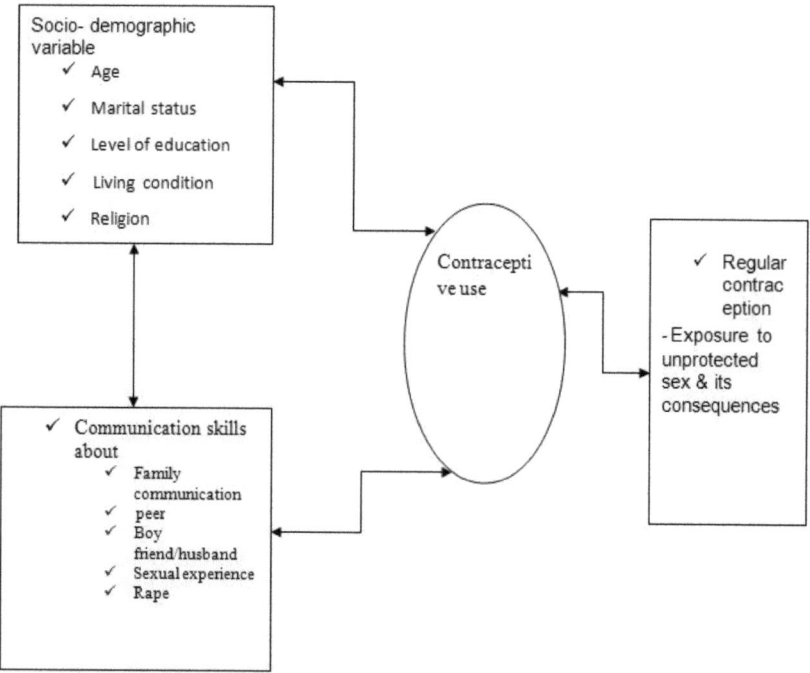

Figure:-1 conceptual formwork of Contraceptive Use and Associated Factors
Source: (review from different literature)

3. Objective

3.1 General Objective

To assess contraceptive use and associated factors among female students in Wolaita Sodo ATVET College, Southern Ethiopia, 2016.

3.2 Specific Objectives

1. To determine contraceptive use among female students in Wolaita Sodo ATVET College.
2. To identify factors associated with contraceptive use among female students in Wolaita Sodo ATVET College.

4. METHODS

4.1 Study Area and Period

This study was conducted with female students in Wolaita Sodo ATVET College located in Soddo. Wolaita Soddo ATVET College is one of the 25 ATVET in Ethiopia. The college has six departments and more than 5000 students in regular, summer and weekend program. The study was conducted from October 21, 2016 to November 9, 2016.

4.2 Study Design:-Institution based cross-sectional study design was used.

4.3 Source Population: - The source population was all female students in Wolaita Sodo ATVET College. The study populations were female students residing on the Wolaita Sodo ATVET College.

4.4 Inclusion criteria: Regular

Exclusion criteria: Summer students, weekend students, night students and those who were not available during the time of questionnaires distribution.

4.5 Sample Size Determination

The sample size was determined using single population proportion formula assuming the proportion of students who are to determine and identified contraceptive use and associated factors is to be 50%. Adding non response rate of 10%, and multiplying by a design effect of 2 due to the multistage nature of the sampling method. The required samples based on the usual formula were as follows:

$$n = \frac{(z\,\alpha/2)^2 p\,(1-p)}{d^2}$$

Where, n=the required sample size

Z= standard score corresponding to 95% confidence interval

P= assumed proportion of aware of students towards the contraceptive.

d= the margin of error (precision) 5%

Then, $n = \frac{1.962 \times (0.5 \times 0.5)}{(0.05)^2} = 384$, from un defined population so, for defined

Population was calculated as follows:

$n = n0$

$(1+n0)$

N Where, no= the sample size from an infinite population.

N= finite population size

n = 384

$N = \dfrac{n}{1+n/N}$

$\dfrac{384}{1+\dfrac{384}{1067}} = \mathbf{282}$

By taking additional 10% contingency for non-response rate, the total sample size was: 282 +10 %(non-response rate) = **310** and considering the design effect of 2x312=**620**

4.6 Sampling Technique/ Procedure

After calculating the sample size, the multistage stratified sampling was employed considering all departments and year of study in the sampling process for the selection of the study subjects.

Initially, of the whole six department three departments, Plant Sciences, Animal Sciences and Natural resources was selected randomly and the total sample size of the study was distributed over each of the department proportional to their size.

In the second stage, including all section from the selected department.Accordingly the sample size of the study allocated to each classes to their size.

Finally, the required numbers of female students were selected randomly (applying SRS) from each year of study again proportional to their size from the randomly selected section.

Sample Size Determination

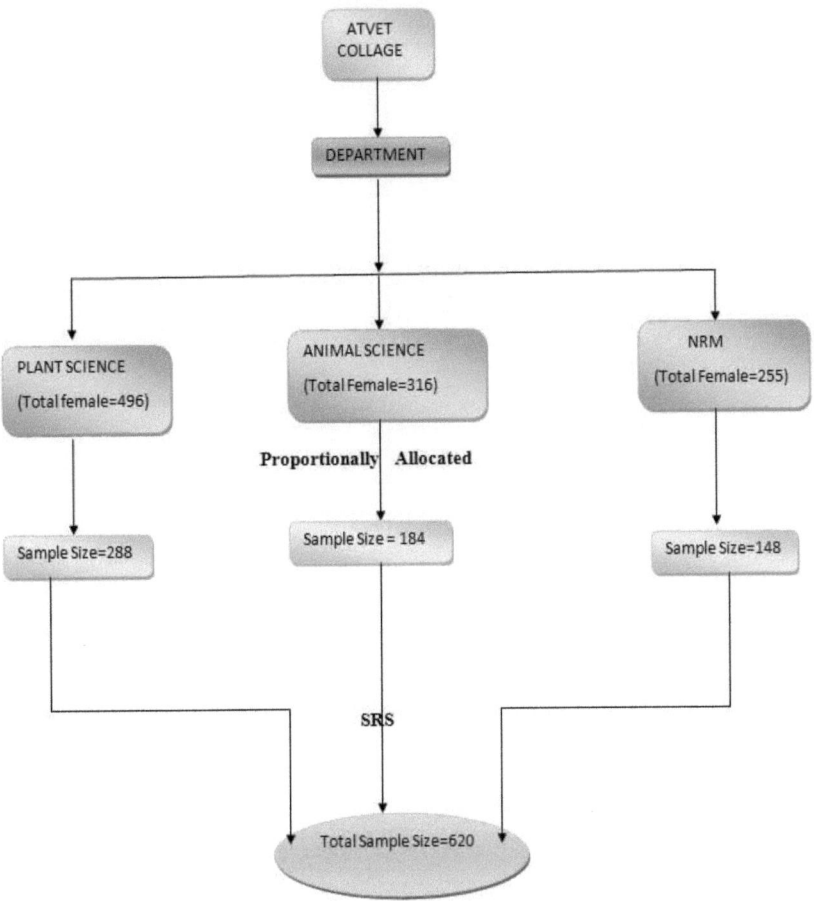

Figure: - 2 Schematic presentation of sample size at waliata sodo ATVET collage, November 2016.

Sample Proportion from Each Section

Natural Science Female Students

➢ 1st year level II- section 1 = $\dfrac{19*148}{255} = 11$

  -section 2 = $\dfrac{21*148}{255} = 11$

  -section 3 = $\dfrac{20*148}{255} = 12$

  -section 4 = $\dfrac{16*148}{255} = 9$

  -section 5 = $\dfrac{17*148}{255} = 10$

  -section 6 = $\dfrac{20*148}{255} = 12$

➢ 1st year level iv —section 1 = $\dfrac{15*148}{255} = 9$

  - section 2 = $\dfrac{18*148}{255} = 10$

  - section 3 = $\dfrac{20*148}{255} = 12$

  - Section 4 = $\dfrac{11*148}{255} = 6$

➢ 2nd year-section 1 = $\dfrac{7*148}{255} = 4$

  -section 2 = $\dfrac{11*148}{255} = 6$

  -section 3 = $\dfrac{13*148}{255} = 8$

➢ 3rd year — section 1 = $\dfrac{12*148}{255} = 7$

  -section 2 = $\dfrac{15*148}{255} = 9$

  -section 3 = $\dfrac{20*148}{255} = 12$

Animal Science Female Students

14

➤ 1st year level ii-section $1= \dfrac{29*184}{316} = 17$

                  -section $2= \dfrac{30*184}{316} = 17$

                  -section $3 = \dfrac{31*184}{316} = 18$

                  -section $4 = \dfrac{30*184}{316} =$

                  -section $5 = \dfrac{28*184}{316} = 16$

➤ 1st year level iv –section $1= \dfrac{18*184}{316} = 11$

                  -section $2= \dfrac{23*184}{316} = 13$

                  -section $3 = \dfrac{21*184}{316} = 12$

➤ 2nd year –section $1= \dfrac{12*184}{316} = 7$

                  -section $2 = \dfrac{13*184}{316} = 8$

                  -section $3 = \dfrac{11* 184}{316} = 7$

➤ 3rd year-section $1= \dfrac{18*184}{316} = 10$

                  -section $2 = \dfrac{20*184}{316} = 12$

                  -section $3 = \dfrac{13*184}{316} = 8$

                  -section $4 = \dfrac{19*184}{316} = 11$

Plant Science Female Students

- 1st year level II - section $1 = \dfrac{27 \times 288}{496} = 16$

  - section $2 = \dfrac{30 \times 288}{496} = 17$

  - section $3 = \dfrac{21 \times 288}{496} = 12$

  - section $4 = \dfrac{23 \times 288}{496} = 13$

  - section $5 = \dfrac{36 \times 288}{496} = 21$

  - section $6 = \dfrac{24 \times 288}{496} = 14$

  - section $7 = \dfrac{25 \times 288}{496} = 14$

- 1st year level iv - section $1 = \dfrac{21 \times 288}{496} = 12$

  - section $2 = \dfrac{27 \times 288}{496} = 16$

  - section $3 = \dfrac{30 \times 288}{496} = 17$

  - section $4 = \dfrac{36 \times 288}{496} = 21$

- 2nd year - section $1 = \dfrac{20 \times 288}{496} = 12$

  - section $2 = \dfrac{18 \times 288}{496} = 10$

  - section $3 = \dfrac{20 \times 288}{496} = 12$

  - section $4 = \dfrac{20 \times 288}{496} = 12$

  - section $5 = \dfrac{20 \times 288}{496} = 12$

- 3rd year - section $1 = \dfrac{22 \times 288}{496} = 13$

  - section $2 = \dfrac{25 \times 288}{496} = 15$

  - section $3 = \dfrac{26 \times 288}{496} = 15$

  - section $4 = \dfrac{25 \times 288}{496} = 15$

4.7 Data Collection Technique

For this study a self administered structured questionnaire was conducted. The questionnaires contain an open as well as closed ended question which covers socio demographic information, and contraceptive use. This was prepared in English and translated to Amharic and then turn to English for its consistency. Well trained data collectors were participated in the data collection process. The study participants was participated based on their willingness in the study. Adequate information was given on how to fill the questionnaire. The principal investigator was made the necessarily supervision and training throughout the data collection period to guide and correct any problems.

The questionnaire was tested before the actual survey within a to ensure its clarity, ordering, consistency and acceptance.

4.8 Study Variables

Dependent Variable: Contraceptive uses by the female students were the dependent variable. **Independent Variables:**

1. Socio-economic educational characteristics.
2. Knowledge of contraceptive methods.
3. Distance from health service site.
4. Family support.
5. Partner or husband opposition.
6. Time convenience for service utilization.
7. Privacy in the delivery of contraceptive services.
8. Confidentiality of client's information regarding contraceptive services.
9. The service provider's approach to delivery.

4.9 Data Quality Management

To assure data quality, data collection tool was prepared after intensive review of relevant literatures from similar studies. Training was give for both data collectors and supervisors concerning on data collection tool for 1 day by the principal investigator. The completeness of the data was checked by data collectors during data collection and also immediately after data collection by the supervisor and principal investigator.

4.10 Data Analysis Procedures

After data collection, each questionnaire was checked for completeness and consistency. The data was analyzed by manually. Then Different frequency tables, graphs and descriptive summaries were used to describe the study variables.

4.11 Ethical Considerations

The proposal was submit to Wolaita Soddo University College of Health Sciences and medicine, School of Public Health, to secure Ethical Clearance. The letter was written from Wolaita Soddo University College of Health Sciences and medicine, School of Public Health to the respective study facilities to enhance the conduct of this study. Informed consent was obtained from individuals selected to be respondents of this study. For this purpose, an information sheet with consent form was attached to each questionnaire which explained about the purpose of the study, confidentiality, and the respondent's full right of voluntary participation. Different measures were taken to assure the confidentiality of study subject's response. Names or any identification was not used.

4.12 Dissemination of the Result

The finding of the study was submitted in a form of a thesis to Wolaita Soddo University College of Health Sciences and medicine, School of Public Health to secure ethical Clearance. The result was publicly defended following submission. Copies were provided to relevant stakeholders.

5. RESULTS

5.1 SOCIO - DEMOGRAPHIC CHARACTERISTICS OF RESPONDENTS

Out of total 1067 female college students 620 were included in the study with a responses rate of 100%. Most of the respondents 328(52.9 %) were within age group of 16-20 years. and ranged from a minimum of 16 years to a maximum of above 30 years. The SD of the survey participants were 1.05919.

Majority of the study subjects 317(51.1%) were from Wolaita ethnic group. And 339(54.7 %) had rural background prior to their entry to the colleges, with the rest being from urban.

With regard to their marital status, about 439(70.8 %) were not currently married, 160(25.8%) were married. Most of the respondents, 490 (79.0 %) were followers of protestant Christianity followed by Orthodox Christianity who accounts 75(12.1 %). **(Table 1)**

Table 1 Socio - demographic and academic characteristics among female college students at Wolaita Soddo ATVET College, November 2016.

Characteristics	No	Percent (%)
Age (years)		
16-20	328	52.9
21-25	133	21.5
26-30	85	13.7
above 30	74	11.9
Total	620	100
Place of origin		
Urban	281	45.3
Rural	339	54.7
Total	620	100
Marital Status		
Single	439	70.8
Married	160	25.8
Widow	21	3.4
Total	620	100
Residence		
In the campus	491	79.2
Out of campus	129	20.8
Total	620	100
Religion		
Orthodox	75	12.1
Muslim	33	5.3
Catholic	11	1.8
Protestant	490	79.0
Others	11	1.8

Total	620	100
Ethnicity		
Wolaita	317	51.1
Gamo	106	17.1
Sidama	94	15.2
Gedyo	20	3.2
Hadya	22	3.5
Other	61	9.8
Total	620	100

5.2 .Prevalence rate of Contraceptive utilization

The survey population were try to investigate on the issues of prevalence of Contraceptive utilization. Based on this the prevalence was (450) 72 % among total female students in walaita sodo ATVET collage.

5.3 FAMILY PLANNING KNOWLEDGE, ATTITUDE & PRACTICES OF THE RESPONDENTS

Family planning knowledge, attitude & practice of the respondents (table 2) showed that, majority of them, 598 (96.5%) of female students in the study had ever heard about regular modern contraceptives. While only 22 students (3.5 %) never heard about any family planning method in their life time. Knowledge of modern contraception 221(35.6%) of respondents knew condom type of contraception, 155(25.0%) oral pill, 149 (24.0 %) Injectable, 44(7.1 %) Norplant, 51 (8.2 %) calendar, type of contraceptive methods. The common sources of information were 152 (24.5 %) from health institution and 115(18.5 %) from mass media. **(Table 2)**

Table 2 Knowledge, attitude and practice about regular type of contraceptives among female College students in Wolaita Soddo ATVET College, November 2016.

Variables	Frequency	Percent (%)
Ever heard about contraceptives		
Yes	598	96.5
No	22	3.5
Total	620	100
Source of information (N598)		
Health institution	152	24.5
Mass media	115	18.5
Friend	146	23.5
Family	124	20.0
Schools	50	8.1
Other	11	1.8
Total	598	100
Know methods of contraceptives		
Condom	221	35.6
Pills	155	25.0
Injectabel	149	24.0
Norplant	44	7.1
Calendar	51	8.2
Total	620	100
Importance of contraception		
Yes	600	96.8
No	20	3.2
Total	620	100
Ever use contraception		
Yes	450	72
No	170	27.4
Total	620	100

Most of the respondents, 600(96.8%) also believed that contraceptives are important in preventing unwanted pregnancy. 450(72 %) of the respondents were ever used contraceptive methods and the most commonly used method was Condom 134 (21.6 %) followed by injecatebl 101 (16.3%). **(Figure 3)**

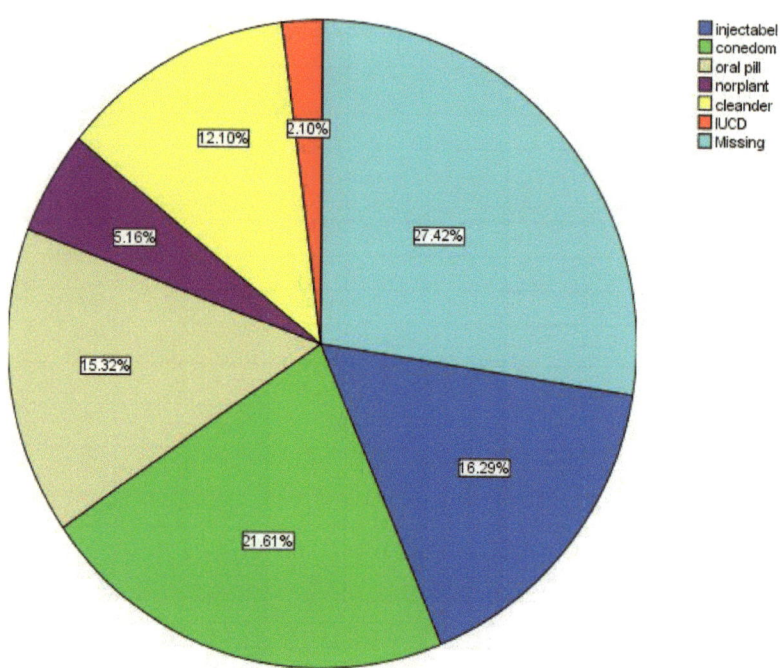

FIGURE 3 - Percentage of type of modern regular contraceptives used by the respondents at waliata sodo ATVET collage, November 2016.

5.4 Contraceptive Practices and Pregnancy Related Characteristics

At the time of the study 357 (57.6%) respondents have ever had not sex in the past. Of those who are sexually active, about 61 (23.1 %) started sex before the age of 18 and 202(76.8%) started sex at 18 years of age and above. Regardless of the respondents having number of sexual partner in their life time, most of them, 190 (72 .2%) had one sexual partner. Concerning rape, respondents who were sexually active in the past, 27(10.3 %) of them were claimed to had sex without their consent or raped.

With regard to pregnancy experience, on those who were sexually active, a total of 69(26.2%) respondents replied that they had been pregnant and with 43(62.3%) gave a history of at least once pregnancy previously. And from the pregnant study subjects, 14(20.2%) had practiced induced abortion. **(Table 3)**

Table 3 – Contraceptive practice and Pregnancy related characteristics among sexually active female college students at Wolaita Soddo ATVET College, November 2016.

Characteristics	No	Percent (%)
Ever had sex (N620)		
Yes	263	42.4
No	357	57.6
Total	620	100
Age at first sex (N263)		
Less than 18	61	23.1
Greater than 18	202	76.8
Total	263	100
Ever had sex without consent or raped (N263)		
Yes	27	10.3
No	236	89.7
Total	263	100
Life time sexual partner(263)		
One	190	72.2
Two	50	19.0
More than 3	23	8.7
Total	263	100
Ever been pregnant (N263)		
Yes	69	26.2
No	194	73.7
Total	263	100
Number of pregnancies (N=69)		

One time	43	62.3
2 time	20	28.9
3 time	6	8.6
Total	69	100
Have induce abortion(N69)		
Yes	14	20.2
No	55	79.7
Total	69	100
Number of induced abortions *(N=14)*		
One time	11	78.5
Two time	2	14.2
More than 3	1	7.1
Total	14	100

5.5 Factors Associated with Contraceptive Use

After analysis, age, religion and time convinces remained associated with contraceptive use. Hence its p-value were < 0.005 where as family support, privacy and confidentiality not associated with the contraceptive use .

Table 4 Factors Associated with Contraceptive Use among Female Students in Wolaita Soddo ATVET College, November 2016.

Variables	Response	Contraceptive use		X^2	P-value
		Yes (%)	No (%)		
Age	16-20	300(48.3)	28(4.5)	8.91	< 0.005
	21-25	112(18)	21(3.3)		
	26-30	74(11.9)	11(1.7)		
	>30	74(11.9)	0		
	Total	560(100)	60(9.6)		
Religion	Orthodox	64(10.3)	11(1.7)	15.07	< 0.005
	Muslim	33(5.3)	0		
	Catholic	11(1.7)	0		
	Protestant	388(62.2)	102(16.4)		
	Other	11(1.7)	0		
	Total	507(100)	113(18.2)		
Family Support		59(9.5)	561(90.4)	0.064	> 0.05
privacy		426(68.7)	194(31.2)	1.271	> 0.05
confidentiality		437(70.4)	183(29.5)	3.032	> 0.05
Time convince		420(67.7)	200(32.3)	16.608	< 0.005

6. Discussion

The contraceptive prevalence rate (CPR) computed in this study was (450) 72%. This CPR was greater than in a study done in northwest Ethiopia in the Dambia district which was 22.5%.

This significant difference may be due to the study populations in two different geographical areas.

The result from this study revealed that greater than two-third (96.5 %) of the respondents had heard of the contraception method. This is greater than the reports on studies in San Francisco (89%). The same is true for the reports from Katmandu- Nepal (68%)[21,26], & Jimma university community high school (64%) [3].

The mean age of respondents of this study was approximately 20 years. Almost near to whole (96.5 %) had ever heard contraceptive pills. The most common source of information was health institution (24.5 %), friend (23.5 %), family (20.0 %), and mass media (18.5%). This showed higher than studies conducted on Uganda, Makerere University among University Students with the mean age of the participants was 21 years and Less than half (45.1%) had ever heard about contraceptive and their most common sources of information about contraceptive were friends (34%), media (24.8%) and schools (19.4%)[10].

Almost half of the total number of our study subjects (57.6 %) reported that they were sexually active in their lifetime with 23.1 % of the respondents had first sex at age below 18 years.

Among the respondents who were sexually active, about 26.2 % become pregnant & of them 62.3 % gave history of at least one pregnancy with 20.2 % had induced abortion. On the other hand, among the total study participants, about 23.1% had first sex at age of below 18 years, 10.3 % ever had sex without their consent, of which 26.2 % were unintended pregnancy, which is higher than studies done in Oromo region, Wolliso town.(3)

After analysis, age, religion and time convinces remained associated with contraceptive use. Hence its p-value was < 0.005 where as family support, privacy and confidentiality not associated with the contraceptive use.

7. LIMITATION OF THE STUDY

7.1 limitation of the study

- Resource constraint in terms of money and time.

-our study design is cross sectional study which is not showing exposure and non exposure out come between contraceptive use and not.

8. CONCLUSION AND RECOMMENDATIONS

8.1 Conclusion

- There is also a need for an intervention of aiming at adolescents' RH issues including contraceptive, by using different Medias as the main means to broadcast appropriate information and Creating Reproductive Health Clubs in the college to address the target issues. ATVET collage clinic also has high contribution on contraceptive utilization by providing access to contraceptive with multiple chooses and enhance the awareness on contraceptive.

8.2 Recommendations

Based on the finding from this study, the following recommendations are forwarded.

-Strategies and programs should be specifically designed to provide appropriate information and access to contraceptive in the country in general and in college institutions in particular to enhance the appropriate awareness of contraceptive among adolescents.

- There is also a need for an intervention of aiming at adolescents' RH issues including contraceptive, by using different Medias as the main means to broadcast appropriate information and Creating Reproductive Health Clubs in the college to address the target issues.

- Similar other studies are recommended to generate more in-depth information on contraceptives.

References

1.   World Health Organization. Programming for adolescent health and development report of WHO/UNFPA/UNICEF study group on programming for adolescents health. Geneva. WHO; 1999.

2.   World Health Organization. Sexual relations among young people in developing countries, evidence from WHO case studies Geneva: 2001

3.   World Health Organization. Making Pregnancy Safer Notes, Volume 1, No.1, October 2008.

4.   United Nations Fund for Population Agency. State of world population 2003: Investing in adolescents' health and rights. *Bulletin.* New York 2003.

5.   United Nations. World population monitoring, Reproductive rights and reproductive health. New York. (2004)

6.   United Nations Fund for Population Agency. The state of world population: The new generation. *Bulletin.* New York 1998.

7.   Central Statistical Agency [Ethiopia] and ICF International. Ethiopia Demographic and Health Survey 2011.Ethiopia and Calverton, Maryland, USA: 2012.

8.   Federal Ministry of Health. National Adolescents and Youth Reproductive Health Strategy (2007-2015), FMOH, 2006..

9.   Ethiopian Central Statistical Authority. National Population Senses Summary Report. CSA 2007.

10.   Mqhayi Mmabatho Margaret, Annsmit Jennifer, Mc Fadyen Margaret Lynn, Beksihiska Mags, Conolly Cathy, Zuma Khangelani and Morroni Chelsea, Misted opportunities contraception Utilization by young South African Women; 2004, African journal of reproductive health 8(2): 137-144.

11.   International Family planning perspectives, estimates of I. abortion in Mexico: what's changed between1996-2006? , December.2008, volume 34, number 4.

12.   Jamieson MA, Hertweck SP, Sanfilippo JS. Contraception: lack of awareness among patients presenting for pregnancy termination. *J Pediatr Adolescent Gynecol.* 1999; 12(1):12–14.

13.   Harrison T. Availability of Family planning: a survey of hospital emergency department staff. *Annals of Emergency Medicine* 2005; 46:105-110.

14.   American College of Obstetricians and Gynecologists. Emergency Contraception. ACOG Practice Bulletin, Number 112. Washington DC: The American College of Obstetrics

and Gynecologists May 2010. To order, call 508-750-8400. Also available in Obstetrics & Gynecology 2010; 115: 1100-1109.

15. Blanchard Kelly, Harrison Tersa, Sello Mosala, Pharmacists; knowledge and perceptions of contraceptive pills in Soweto and the Johannesburg Central Business district South Africa; International family planning perspectives, 2005, 31(4): 172-178.

16. International Consortium for Contraception (ICEC). 2004. Emergency Contraceptive Pills: Medical and Service Delivery Guidelines. Second Edition, the International Consortium for Emergency Contraception, Washington, DC USA.

17. Harrison T. Availability of contraception: a survey of hospital emergency department staff. *Annals of Emergency Medicine* 2005; 46:105-110.

18. Aziken ME, Okonta PI, Ande AB. Knowledge and perception of contraception among female Nigerian undergraduates; International family planning perspectives; June 2003; 29(2):84-87.

19. WHO, UA: global and regional estimates of the incidence of UA and associated mortality in 2003, fifth edition, Geneva: WHO, 2007

20. Wondimu Bekele, Emergency contraceptive: post- secondary school female students' and service providers' perspective (the case of Awassa town), 2008, pp 5-14.

21. Karen Otsea, MPH, Solomon Tesfaye, MD, MPH, Monitoring safe abortion care service provision in Tigray, Ethiopia: Ipas Ethiopia in collaboration with the MOH, Report of a baseline assessment in public-sector facilities, September 2007.

22. Ipas, Children, Youth and Unsafe abortion, 2007, available at: http: /www.iwhc. Org/resources. Accessed on Oct, 2010.

23. Ipas, Children, Youth and Unsafe abortion, 2007, available at: http: /www.iwhc. Org/resources. Accessed on Oct, 2010.

24. Arowojolu A. and Adekunle A, Perception and Practice of Contraceptive by Post-Secondary School Students in South West Nigeria. African Journal of Reproductive Health, 2000, 4(1):56-65.

25. Astede Desta, Contraceptive Knowledge, Attitude and Practice among Bahir Dar University Female Students. Master's thesis in Population Studies submitted to College of Development Studies; Addis Ababa University, 2007.

26. Central Statistical Authority. Ethiopia Demographic Health Survey- 2005. Addis Ababa, Ethiopia. 2006.

27. Berhanu B. Fertility and Contraceptive Use in Rural Dalle, Southern Ethiopia. Ethiopian Journal of HealthDevelopment. 1994; 8(1): 11-21.

28.   Arowojolu A. and Adekunle A, Perception and Practice of Contraceptive by Post-Secondary School Students in South West Nigeria. African Journal of Reproductive Health, 2000, 4(1):56-65.

29.   Friedman S, McQuaid, Grendell J. Current obstetrics & gynecology diagnosis & treatment: 9th Edition; 2003, pp 164-213.

30.   Hu X, Cheng L, Hua X, Glasier A. Advanced provision of Contraceptive to postnatal women in China makes no difference in abortion rates: a randomized controlled trial. *Contraception* 2005; 72:111-116.

31.   Dereje A. assessment of knowledge & practice of EC among female college students in Oremia region south west shewa zone Wolliso town. Gondar university Addis continental institute of MPH unpublished thesis, 2010.

32.   Berhanu D, Assessment of Knowledge Attitude and Practices on Contraceptive among Women Seeking Post Abortion Care in Addis Ababa. Master's thesis in Public Health submitted to the Faculty of Medicine; AAU, 2006.

33.   Wegene T. and Fikre E, knowledge, attitude and practice on emergency contraceptives among female university students in Addis Ababa, Ethiopia, the Ethiopian journal of health development, 2007, volume 21, 112-113.

34.   Keas bury J. Mekbib T. Belay T, Gaym A. Skibiak J. Main streaming EC in Ethiopia's public sector; project results and implication for scale up. Ethiopian journal of RH, 2009; 3(Ec in Ethiopia); 4.

35.   Keas bury J. Mekbib T. Belay T, Gaym A. Skibiak J. Main streaming EC in Ethiopia's public sector; project results and implication for scale up. Ethiopian journal of RH, 2009; 3(Ec in Ethiopia); 4.

Annex- I – Information Sheet

Dear students!

I am now one of the lecturer and researcher in Wolaita Soddo ATVET College Basic sciences' department. I am conducting a survey to assess Contraceptive Use and Associated Factors among Female Students in Wolaita Sodo ATVET College, Southern Ethiopia.

The ultimate purpose of this survey is to collect information necessary for developing programs to prevent unwanted /unplanned pregnancies and its squeals. To attain this purpose your honest and genuine participation is very important and highly appreciable. We, therefore, kindly request you to fill this questionnaire as accurately and carefully as possible. For close ended questions, please encircle your answer and for those you need suggestions write your opinion shortly, precisely &clearly on the space provided for each question.

Please be assured that all the information gathered will be kept strictly confidential and you do not need to write your name or any special identification that might disclose who you are, on any of the questionnaire page. Only the researcher has the access of the information and used it for the study purpose only. You have a full right not to participate in this study.

Data Collector

Name _____ Signature _____ Date

_____

Supervisor

Name _____ Signature _____ Date _____

Annex- II- Consent form

In signing this document, I am giving my consent to participate in the study entitled "assess Contraceptive Use and Associated Factors among Wolaita Sodo ATVET College Female Students, Southern Ethiopia,''.

I have been informed that the purpose of this research project and I understand that I am selected to participate in this study randomly. I have been informed that my participation in this study is willing full and voluntary even I have right to refuse or interrupt the filling of questionnaire and my name will not be mentioned on the questionnaire.

I, undersigned, have understood the purpose of the study & fully agree to participate in the study.

Signature of the participant------------------ Date ------------------------

Thank you, have a nice day!

Annex II Questionnaire

Section - I - Socio- demographic characteristics and factor related with contraceptive of the respondents.

Q.No_	Question	Responses coding categories	Skip to
Q.01	How old are	1.16-20 2.21-25 3.26-30 4.>30	
Q.02	Where did you come from?	1.Urban 2.Rural	
Q.03	Tell me about your current Marital status?	1.Single 2.Married 3.Divorced 4.Widowed	
Q.04	Where do you live now?	1.In campus 2.Outside campus	
Q.05	If your response to Q.04 is #2 with whom do you live now?	1.With parent 2.With peers in rental house 3.Alone in rental house 4.With boy friend 5.With husband 6.If other specify_____	
Q.06	What is your Religion?	1.Orthodox 2.Muslim 3.Catholic 4.Protestant 5.Other, specify_____	
Q.07	What is your ethnicity?	1.Wolaita 2.Gamo 3.Sidama 4.Gedeyo 5.Hadya 6.Other, 7.other specify_____	
Q.08	Which year are you attending now?	1.First year 2.Second year 3.Third year	

32

Section - II- on contraception and factor related with it

Q.09	Have you ever heard about Family Planning Methods?	1.Yes 2.No	If no skip to Q.09
Q.10	If you say yes for Q. 09 where did you get the information?	1.Health institution 2.Mass media 3.Friend 4.Family 5.School 6.Other, specify _____	
Q.11	Which one method of contraception do you know? (more than one response is possible)	1.Condom 2.Oral pill 3.Injectables 4.Norplant 5.Calendar 6.IUCD 7.Other, specify _____	
Q.12	Do you believe that family planning methods Prevent pregnancy?	1.Yes 2.No	
Q.13	Do you think that contraceptive is important?	1.Yes 2.No	
Q.14	Have you ever used any type of contraceptive?	1.Yes 2.No	
Q.15	If you say yes for Q.14, which method do you use?(multiple is possible)	1.Injectable 2.Condom 3.Oral pill 4.Norplant 5.Calendar 6.IUCD	
Q.16	Have you ever had sexual intercourse?	1.Yes 2.No	
Q.17	Have you ever happened sex without your consent?	1.Yes 2.No	
Q.18	If your response is yes for Q,# 17 who forced you to have sex?	1.Student/ friend 2.Teacher 3.Relative in the parent 4.Un known person 5.Other, specify_____	

Q.19	What problem you faced after the forced sex?	1.Unwanted pregnancy 2.STI 3.Tension 4.Nothing at all 5.Other, specify_____	
Q.20	If you face un wanted pregnancy, how did you solve the problem?	1.I continued pregnancy& gave birth 2.Induced abortion by different means's 3.I go to health institution 4.Other, specify_____	
Q.21	At what age were you had the first sexual intercourse?	1.Below 18 years old 2.18 years and above 3.I don't remember	
Q.22	How many partners have you ever had for sexual intercourse up to date?	1.One 2.Two 3.More than three 4.I don't remember them	
Q.23	Have you ever been pregnant?	1.Yes 2.No	
Q.24	If 'Yes', how many times?	_____	
Q.25	Have you ever practiced induced abortion?	1.Yes, of course 2.No, I don't	
Q.26	If yes for Q#25, how many times?	_____	
Q.27	Do you intend to use contraceptive method to avoid unwanted pregnancy in the future?	1.Yes 2.No 3.May be	
Q.28	What are factors related with your use of contraception use	Age------- 1.yes 2.no Religion------ 1.yes 2no Family support --1.yes 2.no Partner opposition…1.yes 2.no Privacy ……1.yes 2.no Confidentiality…1yes 2.no Time convince 1.yes 2no	

YOUR KNOWLEDGE HAS VALUE

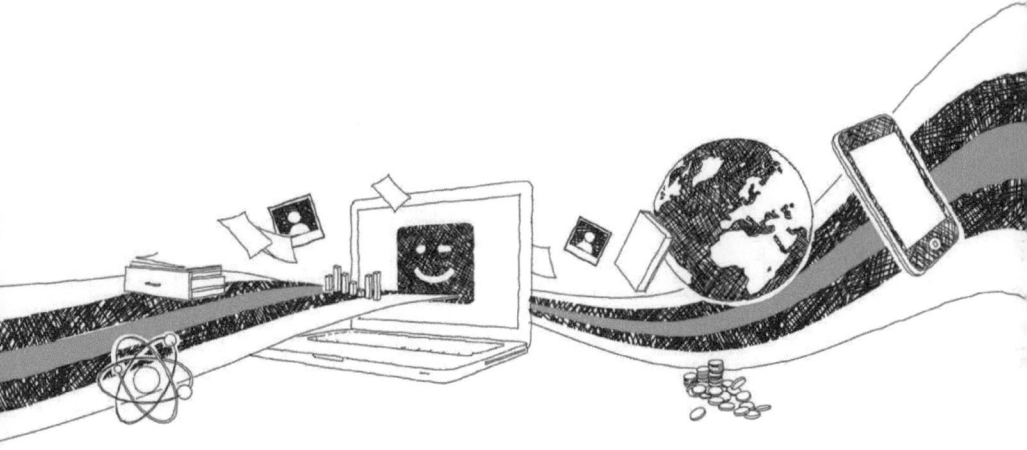

- We will publish your bachelor's and
  master's thesis, essays and papers

- Your own eBook and book -
  sold worldwide in all relevant shops

- Earn money with each sale

Upload your text at www.GRIN.com
and publish for free

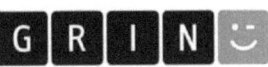